How To Meet And Bang A MILF

A Guide to MILF's, Cougars and Mid Age Women

Written By:
Eddie Chaffin

Eddie Chaffin Books
Copyright 2011

This book contains adult language and narratives not intended for children under the age of eighteen or the weak of heart.

All rights reserved. No part of this book may be reproduced by any means whatsoever without the written permission from the author, except brief portions quoted for purpose of review.

All information in this book has been carefully researched and checked for factual accuracy. However, the author and publisher make no warranty, express or implied, that the information contained herein is appropriate for every individual, situation, or purpose, and assumes no responsibility for errors or omissions. The reader assumes the risk and full responsibility for all actions, and the author will not be held responsible for any loss or damage, whether consequential, incidental, and special or otherwise that may result from the information presented in this publication.

Contact Eddie at:
EddieChaffin@rocketmail.com

Table of Contents

Introduction..4
The Difference's Between a Young Woman and a M.I.L.F..5
The First Tip 8
What You Need to Know 10
Cougar and M.I.L.F Online Dating Sites..15
How to Sexually Please and Bang a M.I.L.F..17
My Two True Stories..21

Introduction

M.I.L.F. No, we are not talking about The Moro Islamic Liberation Front which is located in the southern Philippines; that is an Islamic militant group you fool!

We are talking about very beautiful and sexy creatures known to man that are women in the age range of thirties and forties, fifties and very seldom, sixties (depending how desperate the male is), and they just might be a mother as well. I believe when you start looking at women that are 60 and up you're hitting granny territory and your second head may be suffering from a hangover. The true acronyms for M.I.L.F are Mothers I'd Like to Fuck. If it was up to me, the acronyms would be M.I.L.F.H. Mothers I'd Like to Fuck Hard! The "H" would be silent of course.

In all actuality, a M.I.L.F doesn't need to be a mother at all. Oh, no no, she can just be a very attractive thirty five, forty five or fifty five year old woman who never given birth to a child in her life. Hell, this type of M.I.L.F might just have a tighter pussy than the women who did give birth whose vaginas look like they've been hit by a freight train. I know; I have been there! There is no pleasure in a train tunnel guys!

So, from a guy with experience dating M.I.L.F's, as well as having banged them all, I, Eddie Chaffin, will guide you through my book on the DO's and DON'T's, the HOW's and HOW nots, STEPS and TIPS about courting the M.I.L.F or COUGAR of your desire, and HOW to make love to them.

However I do not offer any guarantees because it's hard to know if you practice self hygiene or not. Straight up tip number one guys, women do not like the smell of sweaty balls, and for sure do not like the smell of sweaty balls smacking them in the face. So take that shower before making any attempts or thinking about finding a M.I.L.F !

Now don't get me wrong, this book is not only intended for men, but also for the women out there that enjoy the taste of another woman's sweet honey just as much!

Also, after my guidance and tips I will share a couple true stories of mine towards the end of this book - and only in this book. But please look for my other books I will be producing in the near future. It will be true sex stories and fiction sex stories about M.I.L.F's, just to get you M.I.L.F lovers revved up!

"Men, start your engines!"

The Difference's Between a Young Woman and a M.I.L.F

I remember when I was a teenage boy in the 80's, way before the term was coined "M.I.L.F" I had a strong attraction and infatuation about making love or banging a women in her thirties or forty's. I didn't care if she had kids or not; that was the age I wanted and wanted desperately. I was not at all attracted to girls my age or even in their twenties; she had to be between thirty to fifty years of age. I was only thirteen or fourteen when I first started this fantasy of mine, a fantasy still alive today. Women of this age are mature in nature, mentally, physically and sexually. Majority of girls age twenty nine and under are still naïve, immature, and sure the hell don't know if they want sex or not. Mid age women know what they want, and they want sex!

Come on guys, have you ever dated a girl in her teens or twenties before? What's the first thing they tell you? "I shouldn't, or I'm still a virgin, I can't". Their hormones are not fully activated yet, unlike a mid age woman or a M.I.L.F. Do not waste your time with these young females; a lot of them will only get you into trouble.

You say what kind of trouble? Ok here are just a few.

1) If you have sex with a girl under twenty nine, there is a much higher probability that she will feel guilty the next day from this forbidden act she just committed. Even if she gave you the ok for penetration and says something stupid like "pull out before cumming in me." But the next day she may slap a rape charge against your stupid ass. You must then prove it was consensual at the time. I never had this experience but I sure can tell you this, it would be very hard to prove your innocence and the judge always favor the female of these types of cases 2 to 1! This inexperienced young girl just ruined your life! You damn idiot! (Excuse my bluntness).

2) Girls in their teens and twenties are not mature enough mentally or responsible enough to stay on birth control. They always forget to take the damn pill! But a mid age or M.I.L.F is more responsible. Secondly, in most cases your M.I.L.F has had her tubes tied. I tell you what guys, there is nothing more exciting than being able to release a full load into your lady and never worry about her getting pregnant.

So you do decide to have sex with a young girl (a girl under 29) and you didn't pull out like she wanted. She may come to you in a few weeks with the news that you are a new daddy. Not unless you're ready to take care of a kid for the next eighteen years, this young immature girl just ruined your life! You damn idiot!

You know I should write a book directed at guys dating young girls and call it "You Damn Idiot!" What do you think?

Are you getting my drift here yet? Girls under 29 are not worth the fucking! Pretend they don't exist. There are plenty of mid age women or M.I.L.F's out there!

Ok, here is a third reason not to date a girl under 29:

3) They usually still have a curfew! I am damn serious. Most girls today still live with mommy and daddy. I remember when I was young and one of the very few times I gave girls my own age a chance, (I mean how else would I know all this shit?), I was 26 and she was 26, I met her and asked her out. I kid you not; she wanted me to go meet her fuckin parents so they can determine if she could go out with me that night, and on top of that, she could only stay out till 10 pm! I literally felt like a two hour babysitter!
If you're not laughing your ass off at this, then you have no sense of humor!

I believe this is why the acronym M.I.L.F was invented, for men like me. If you feel a strong urge to be with a mid age woman, children or not, you are by far not alone. For I stand along side you. I believe that in the old days, like the days of your grandparents and great grandparents, girls under twenty nine were by far more mature in everything (mentally and sexually) than that same age group as today. Let me explain:

Back in the 1800's and early 1900's, girls as young as sixteen or fifteen were marring men in their mid twenties. I kid you not! Example are my own grandparents, my grandfather was 25 when he proposed to my grandmother at age 16. They have been married ever since; fifty some years today. You see times were different; it was hard to make a living (harder than today) so young girls were mature enough to decide the fact that it would be easiest for all families if they were to marry. This in a sense forced girls to grow up faster mentally. My grandmother was working the farm and helping her parents pay the mortgage at age thirteen! You don't see girls paying rent today at that age, hell not even at age 29!

Today, if you see young girls living independently (particularly around 20 yrs old) don't be fooled that it's their own hard wages paying for that rent. Ninety percent of the time their daddy is paying their rent, and paying it through their twenties! Don't be fooled by these young girls that are trying to put on the illusion that they are living independently. Little do you know daddy's name is on the rental contract and on the car's title.

Society in the last few decades has morphed this age bracket (girls between 18 and 29) into a completely new breed of whiners and unworthy girls. If you are still not getting the picture turn on your TV to that reality show where it shows teens and early twenties girls getting pregnant and having babies. Have you noticed their adolescent behavior? Their spoiled and moody attitudes? Why would a man in his right mind ever want that? If you do, than you are a sick man for sure. Time to get both heads examined!

The First Tip

Most men love mid age women (as myself) that have children or not (I'm talking about mothers who had that train tunnel tightened up a bit). So when a man speculates that a mid age lady standing next to him in a line at the grocery store may be a mother as well, he is immediately aroused even more with a possible hard on. The maturity and age of this lady is a turn on that is very hard to turn off, if ever.

In chapter one, I was speaking about the invention of the new found movement of M.I.L.F. Have you noticed that M.I.L.F came into existence at the turn when girls under 29 became so unreliable and untrustworthy? It was like at the same time! Men grew tired of these young girls and what they had become, so a new evolution was formed to fill that space: M.I.L.F. You ever hear the term "Out of necessity Comes Invention or Creativity"? M.I.L.F was a new necessity for what young women had taken away or no longer is; Pure and simple.

Remember the example I had given about my grandparents? My grandmother was a very mature young lady at age sixteen, thus attracting my grandfather at age 25; and I don't think my grandfather would have dated anybody under 29 in today's society.

Maybe one day the M.I.L.F movement will die, but only after the young women reach maturity. I doubt that will ever happen. Something else to take note of: through all the ages of mankind M.I.L.F did not come into existence until shortly after the feminist movement. Hmmm, does the feminist movement have something to do with young girls behaving like the way they do today which is a turn off to men? Possibly the answer is yes.

Perhaps the feminist movement is what caused the M.I.L.F movement? I'm not certain, but the dots do connect. Here is the truth: when a woman exhibits feminist liberal traits to me, it's a major turn off; and I do know that feminist attitudes are much higher in woman under age 29! Boy, do I love connecting dots!

Here we are talking all about M.I.L.F's, but we have hardly mentioned another well-known term: "COUGARS". There is a reason that certain type of mid age women are called cougars; they are like a cougar in bed, and sometimes they may do a cougar roar for you during sex. They are instantly attracted to young men! A M.I.L.F can be a cougar for sure. Let's use these two terms interchangeably through out the book.

#1 Strategy to getting a sexy cougar, mid age woman or even a M.I.L.F. is...
Consistency.

Too many times will a guy searching for a Cougar end up with a shattered ego because he was denied the first time. Feeling burned he will never attempt again.

Put that shy guy in the closet and learn to take the NO's with out getting hurt by it.
I know the feeling of denial. I have had more denials and NO's than YES's from cougars and M.I.L.F.s in my life!

Consistency is the key. Start looking at your NO's from a Cougar or M.I.L.F as one more step to that YES! That's what I did years ago and I have had dozens of Cougars and M.I.L.F's in the last ten years! So, I had dozens of Cougars or m.i.l.f's but also hundreds of denials. When a mid age woman said NO to me, it made me happy because I knew I was one step closer to getting my Cougar or M.I.L.F.

Remember the hunter hunting deer in the woods; this hunter hunts for one solid week. Day after day he either misses a shot (representing a denial) or he just never came across a deer. But his consistency paid off on that 7th day! He shot a beautiful deer and took her home! Guys, that deer is your M.I.L.F or Cougar you been dreaming about and is now in the flesh for your desires.

Women in this age group are much hornier than a girl under 29 years of age; true fact! Here is another fact, Cougars are always found at speed dating groups! Forget hitting on Mrs. Jones at the local gym; (by the way women hate that, so why piss her off?) cougars can always be found at speed dating groups. Look one up in your area.

Here is your assignment...

Keep a journal of your no's and yes's with dates on it, by doing this you will soon see the formula and you will be able to master the system.

Next write down the changes that you need to make to match the consistency plan I wrote about.

Write down your goals on paper, what you want and when you want it. This will give you the motivation to go after it!

What You Need to Know

Believe it or not, there are a lot of men out there that are *not* looking for a younger woman. While at one time the idea may have been taboo, it's increasingly becoming socially accepted and a popular practice. According to the US Census, 12 percent of marriages involve younger men and older women.

As a matter of fact, classic funny gal Lucille Ball was six years older than her husband Desi Arnez. Audrey Hepburn was seven years older than Robert Wolders.

Pop music icon Madonna was ten years older than Guy Ritchie and Elizabeth Taylor was twenty years older than Larry Fortensky. It may be hard for some people to understand why some men are drawn to older women, but more often than not, it has to do with the compatibility of two personalities.

One theory is that older women tend to be more mature and can better handle a serious relationship. Often times, they are better equipped to deal with situations than a woman in her twenties. They have more life experience, both emotionally and sexually. Others speculate that it's a man's natural tendency to search for a mate that reminds him of his mother.

For the men that become involved in this kind of situation, it can become a tangled mess. Friends and family may give you a hard time. Some may embrace it, but chances are, many will continue to ridicule your relationship. Here are some tips to make things work:

A relationship with an older woman is likely to be an honest one. A mature woman has no problem speaking her mind and is absolutely sure of what she wants. Don't be afraid to speak your mind too. Talk to her about what you're looking for. If you're only looking for some fun and company, then let her know. It's best to set things straight before things go too far.

Remember, an older woman is independent. This includes finances. Older women that are looking for a younger man tend to be successful businesswomen, or hold high positions at large corporations. When she demands to pay her way, don't get offended, or see this as emasculating. Older women hold their emotional and financial independence in the highest regard. However, it wouldn't be a bad idea to surprise her with a home-cooked meal, or a surprise getaway at your expense. She'll find the gesture to be sweet and thoughtful. Just because she's older, doesn't mean she's not still a woman.

Do you loathe the social obligations that come along with seeing a younger woman? All of those family gatherings, holidays, endless dinner dates and constant phone calls can be more than what you bargained for. Older women are ferociously independent and will allot time for their career, family and friends. Her life will not revolve around you and you'll more than likely be pushed to the back burner. You need to be ready for this.

There's no nonsense with older women. They know what they want, and they will speak their mind. They're not afraid to tell you what they want in a relationship, or in bed. This keeps the trivial arguments to a minimum and leaves more room for fun. With an older woman, you won't have to deal with the games younger women play. Rather than saying one thing, and meaning another, she'll usually tell it like it is. There may be times when she'll be flaky, or vague, but for the most part, older women like to keep things simple and straightforward. They've been there, done that and are, frankly, over it.

Did you know that women don't reach their sexual peak until they're in their late 30s into their 40s? Men reach theirs while they're in their 20s! There's a good chance that an older woman and a younger man will be compatible in bed. Don't automatically assume this will be the case, as great sex has many other factors. However, because older women don't have the emotional anxiety that women in their twenties have, the probability is higher that it will be great.

So, what exactly is so appealing about cougars? While many of them are divorced, they are usually fit, confident and financially independent women. What's not to love? Younger men (often called cubs) that are looking for a mature women who are secure, genuine and can carry on a conversation, will find a cougar alluring.

Cougars will make use of internet dating sites, clubs and bars to find their cubs. Most people perceive cougars as older women that prey on younger, gullible men. Some cougars are only interested in one night stands, but there are plenty looking for more than just a fling.

Young men will often get agitated when they talk to women under the age of 29 because they're usually uncertain of themselves and giggle quite a bit. On top of what's already been discussed, there are so many more benefits to cougar dating. The idea of dating a man who's younger is thrilling to a cougar. To be fancied by a younger, attractive and passionate man that would normally be off limits, is a huge turn on. Plus, there's no need for Viagra.

A mature woman, who is just looking to have fun, rather than settle down, would find cougar dating appealing. She and her cub can enjoy their time together and then move on without any strings attached. For a young man who has plans to start a family someday, this is the ideal relationship. The two get to have fun together and learn from each other. Any new experiences can be used to positively affect any future relationships.

Be sure to protect your heart while dating a M.I.L.F., however. If the sex is amazing, the two of you laugh a lot, and your conversations are open and honest, it can be very easy for feelings to get involved. It's okay if both of you fall for each other, but when it only happens to one person, it can be heartbreaking. To be the one who's more invested emotionally, can be devastating.

The bottom line is: M.I.L.F.s and Cougars are likely to break your heart. If you really want to get involved with a M.I.L.F. or Cougar, watch your emotions and don't let yourself fall for her right away. You'll see that most of the cougars out there are only looking to have sex with a hard stud.

When younger men date older women, their friends can have an impact on the relationship. The larger the gap in age, the more problematic it can become. A man who's in his twenties will have very different friends than a woman in her fifties. Chances are they're not going to have much in common.

There are always exceptions to the rule, but it's not likely that both groups of friends will get along perfectly. If there's no common ground between either group, it becomes hard for everyone to get together. One option is to come to an agreement on only seeing one group of friends at a time. This, however, makes hosting any kind of party or other special occasion a problem, as you have to exclude a certain group of friends. Sure, the two of you see no problem with the age difference, but your friends may find it awkward to spend time with an older crowd.

Even though relationships between younger men and older women are more well received now than in the past, you will still encounter people who are not as welcoming to the idea. Keep in mind that your relationship could bring forth unpleasant comments or opinions from family, friends, and strangers.

Because of this, you'll need to have some thick skin to deal with these remarks and unsolicited advice from others.

If you're going to get involved with an older woman, don't be naive. Understand she's going to have some hefty baggage. What single person in their 40s wouldn't? Be prepared for her to have ex-husbands, ex-boyfriends, children, divorces, debt, and work pressures.

If you're going to get romantically involved with an older woman, you have to be willing and ready to accept this. You won't necessarily deal with these issues, but they'll be prevalent in her life and she's going to have a lot more to deal with than a women in her early 20s.

Keep in mind that when you get involved with an older woman, you're going to have to deal with people like your boss or parents, ridiculing you for your decision. But to your friends, you'll be a hero! They'll be pleading for you to tell them what it's like to have sex with a Cougar or M.I.L.F.

Either way, there's going to be a lot of talk. Maybe you're one of those guys who likes all of the attention, or are secure enough in the relationship to go ahead with it.

Older women are usually fresh divorcees, and are just looking to have a good time. She doesn't want to get involved in a serious relationship; she just wants to find a man to have fun with.

A younger guy with no attachments and plenty of stamina is easily able to satisfy all of her needs. Being with an older woman will definitely teach you a thing or two in the bedroom. She'll have no sexual inhibitions, she'll know exactly what she wants, and will probably have a few tricks of her own.

An older, more mature woman will have the confidence that comes from life experience. She'll be self-assured and able to handle any curve ball that life throws at her. Like everyone else, she's bound to have a bad day or two. But her bad days are probably because of something more than just a broken nail or bad hair day.

At the end of the day, it's all on you to decide if this kind of relationship is right for you. Weigh the pros and cons. I know, the idea of having incredible sex with a confident, mature woman, with no strings attached, is a tough decision.

AARP conducted a survey back in 2003 which showed 35% of single women aged 50 and over, felt the baggage men their age carried was their biggest complaint. Most cougars want to talk about and do new, exciting things, not reminisce about the past. A younger man can provide her with the thrill she's looking for, without having to deal with an ex-wife and kids.

Nancy D. O'Reilly, a clinical psychologist, makes the claim, "Older women are confident, sexually mature, they don't have inhibitions, they know what they like, and they know what they want." In other words, older women are simply looking for companionship and a commitment-free sexual relationship.

When you're talking about the relationship between an older woman and a younger man, the word "dating" also includes one-night stands, flings and longstanding commitments. Keep in mind that that U.S. Census statistic of 12% of marriages being between younger men and older women insinuates that a lot of the non-marital links are purely for sex and fun.

Cougar and M.I.L.F Online Dating Sites

An online dating site dedicated to cougars is not really like any of the normal matchmaking websites. The cougar dating websites work in two different ways: They're either going to match an older woman with a younger man, or they're going to match a younger man with an older woman. With a cougar dating site, you can specify whether you are looking to just find a friend, have fun, or a long lasting relationship. They'll also have blogs, forums, chat rooms, and messaging systems, on top of the usual dating site features. What's great about cougar dating sites is that men and women are able to talk to each other in the privacy of their homes.

Because more and more people are starting to accept both internet dating and the "cougar/cub" relationship, the trend is continuing to grow. There was a time when internet dating was seen as unsafe, or a sign of desperation. Now, it's one of the most popular forms of dating. If you're looking to find a cougar, using an internet dating site can help you cross that generational divide slowly. This is just one more reason this trend will continue to thrive.

The web, along with all of its dating sites, is a perfect place to start while looking for a M.I.L.F. Decide exactly what it is you want: race, height, hair color, eye color, etc. The biggest problem is figuring out how to approach a cougar online. You definitely don't want to be turned away when you make the move to first and second base.

If you can learn a straightforward, step-by-step process to use when you make your very first contact, you'll have an advantage that most guys only dream they had. Learn what women want to hear, how to ask for her personal e-mail, or phone number.

The first impression is everything! Your opening e-mail is your first impression. Don't start by saying "Sup?" or "Wow, you're hot!" when you first contact her. Remember, this is an older woman, so try to think about how she wants to be approached. Try to be more mature and sophisticated.

Start by introducing yourself to her and explain why you're contacting her. What was it about her that caught your attention? Include some information about yourself as well.

You can try breaking the ice with a joke, so she can get some sort of idea what your personality is like. Keep in mind that this is your first impression. Your humor should be clean. You don't know her and you don't want to offend her in any way.

Be sure to ask her questions about herself. Try asking about something you read on her profile, as this will show her you really read through it. This way, your potential mate knows you're interested and want to get to know her more.

If the woman has a picture, but you don't, you're wasting your time by contacting her. Having to ask you for your photo is going to really put her off. You obviously want to see her, so you can expect that she wants to see you too.

Speak to her like an adult. This is not a text message to one of your friends, so refrain from using any IM language. In fact, use capitalization when it calls for it. If your e-mail looks like one long text message, she may just turn you away because you don't seem smart enough for her. Save the text messages for later, if she's okay with that.

Do your homework. Find out the differences between what young women want and older women anticipate. An older woman is going to expect a mature introduction and a photo. They're looking for a fun, open-minded and appealing man. Having an understanding of these things will get you far with a beautiful, older woman.

Remember, a cougar has been on the dating scene longer than you have. Cougars have a lot more experience with sex and relationships. They know exactly what it is they want. Be mindful of both your and your mate's needs. Be crystal clear about whether or not the relationship is going to be exclusive. Don't play hard to get with an older woman. It doesn't work. She expects her man to be there when she needs him, to be passionate and willing to give her all of his attention, whenever she craves it.

How to Sexually Please and Bang a M.I.L.F

Ok, so you mastered the technique in meeting a m.i.l.f and you have a mid-age woman at your pad. What are you doing next? Well, for starters get rid of your obvious nervous look! This will turn any woman of maturity off!

Here are few simple and important rules to follow:

If she hasn't given you sex by the third date, I say dump her. She has no intentions mating with you anytime soon. If you do have sex, wrap your dick until you been with her for a while, so you can get a feel if she is two timing you; this will help you know for sure if she is clean of any diseases.

Never kiss her on the first date, but do ask for a second date. On this second date, you make the advance, lean in and kiss her lips. If she doesn't want it, you should be able to read her vibes if you are intuitive. If she is reluctant kissing you, don't ask her on a third date. Start from scratch.

If a M.I.L.F wants sex on the first date or night of meeting you, no matter how tempting, don't do it!

She may be a slut! I guarantee she has some kind of venereal disease. Stay away from one night stands; it will burn you for life!

This is a true story: a good friend of mine found a beautiful M.I.L.F, and on the first night and he ate her pussy out. After a week, his mouth and lips developed boils that leaked puss! It took him weeks to get rid of it.

Also, if her pussy has a strong fish odor, zip up and run! Although that smell could mean anything, such as she never douches or doesn't ever wash down there, but it could also mean there has been too many men down there recently. Too many loads by different men will create a cesspool like condition inside her slimy vagina. Yikes!!

Ok, enough rules for right now, lets get back to how a guy should sexually please a M.I.L.F or Cougar. After the second or third date, you two are at your place for a nightcap. Start strategizing in your head when and how you will kiss her. Believe it or not, women can tell if you will be good in bed just by your kiss alone. Don't ever give pecks on the lips; you are not kissing your mother here! Tilt your head to the side, put your lips to hers and kiss. Slightly open your mouth to give her indication you want to tongue. If she remains tight lip, then she may not be the type who likes to French Kiss, so don't push it. If on the other hand she opens and accepts your tongue, meet yours with hers, tip to tip first. Don't force it down her throat!

By now, you will know by her vibes if she wants more. If she is enjoying the kiss slightly move your hand up to her breast. Only cup one breast, don't be a moron and try to handle both with only one hand, you will look stupid!

Squeeze that breast ever so gently; give it a little massage, even through her shirt. If she hasn't taken your hand off her breast at this point, keep rubbing it.

If by chance she takes your hand off her breast, end the make out session right then and there, tell her you apologize and walk her out the front door. She has no intentions having sex with you. You are now wasting your good time. Keep in mind this should be on the second or third date.

Ok, you are making great strides now. She is freely allowing you to rub her breast. Good Job so far! At this point your dick should be hard as a rock. Keep in mind, her being an experienced woman will know this; it is also very hard to hide a solid hard cock from a woman of this caliber.

Depending on the shirt she is wearing, your next move is to make skin to skin contact with her breast. If she is wearing a button down shirt, you must take both hands and start unbuttoning that blouse from top down. After unbuttoning it, take it up off over her shoulders then down her arms. If she has a pull over shirt, slip both hands under and firmly hold both breasts, then use both hands to take her shirt up over her head, not fast, but soft and gentle.

You must understand this, for some reason women love to be undressed by the male. It's a sexual thing.

Most women are scared of their body's appearance in bright light; ask her at this point if she would like the lights dimmed or a candle lit. This way it won't make her feel uncomfortable. If she wants a candle or the lights down, then do it. A later sex encounter is when you request to have more lighting, after she is comfortable with you, but not now!

She is now in her bra, do not gawk at her breast; it will be a turn off to her. Instead reach around and unstrap her bra. Now this can be a difficult task for beginners. I myself can do it with one hand in no time. For the beginner, as you reach around her back feel for the straps and where they connect. Place your left hand on the left strap and vice versa the other hand. What you are going to do is grip the straps where they connect and then bring your hands together while firmly holding the straps. This should unfasten the bra.

Practice does make perfect, so if you don't want to look like a buffoon, I suggest getting a bra and practicing the unclasping part. I don't care where you get the damn bra, find a way and practice on it. Just don't tell your friends, they may think you are a cross dresser!

After her bra is off, her breasts will be before you in their full glory. This is the time you will rub her nipples and areoles. Do not pinch or squeeze them hard, they are sensitive. Play with them a bit; this is when foreplay really starts. Play with them, rub them and go down for a few licks, kisses and tenderly suck her nipples. Don't suck hard or she may yell.

So, between kissing her mouth, kissing and sucking her breast, she should be getting wet. This is when you unstrap her pants and pull them down and off her feet. Usually the man does not take off the shoes, she will do this. Women are usually afraid of showing off their feet barefoot. But if she asks for you to take them off, then do it.

At this point she is in her panties only. She also should be flat on her back. Do not be too fast slipping her panties off! Use this time to foreplay a bit. Start at her mouth and keep kissing her and tonguing her if she permits. Go back to her breast and lick the nipples again. Use long strokes with your tongue around the curves of her breast. Lightly suck the nipples a bit. Squeeze the nipples a bit, but ever so gently.

Start kissing her tummy area, and keep kissing along the way to her hips. Use your tongue and lick her hips and thighs a bit. Take this moment and pass over her vagina that is still under the panties. Take a few good smells as you pass over from hip to hip. This will help give you any indicators if she smells like fish or not. If the smell is abundant, don't go any further.

If you do not smell rotten fish by now keep the foreplay going. Lick down her legs a bit, and then back up to her thighs. Kiss along the way as well. During this foreplay, you must compliment her of her body; tell her how wonderful her skin smells and how good her skin taste.

Put both hands on her thighs and slide them up till you reach her panties, this is the moment you will slowly take them down. After they are off, keep up the foreplay, kissing and licking her hips and legs. Do a few more over passes from hip to hip and smell for any fish. Go back up to her breast to do a few more sucks and licks.

Meet back with her face to face and keep kissing her. In the mean time place your leg between her two legs and use it as a wedge to pry her legs gently open. As she opens her legs more, you will be placing both legs between her legs now. At this moment, you should be hip to hip with her. You can do one of two things at his moment, one is take your finger and reach down to her pussy lips, and start fingering her clit, or you can quickly take your pants off get back into position and ever so gently put the head of your cock up to her clit. Do not insert yet! You must grip your cock and rub that head in a circular motion on her clit for a while.

After a little bit of playing with her clit with your dick head, slowly insert it into her vagina and feel the warmth. Pump her for a while; never cum early. If you feel the urge to cum you must practice the technique and hold back. Early ejaculation is a turn off to M.I.L.F's and Cougars.

One of many techniques I use to hold early ejaculation, is I put my mind immediately in a different spot, like work. Any place that is not sexually exciting. After I lose the urge to cum, I get right back to it. You should always make sure she cums first, then you can have your fun. Women are strange that way, if they feel that you cummed before them and then you stop fucking her, she will think you only wanted one thing: to please yourself only.

During this first encounter, use your sniffer indiscreetly for fish smells; you can always stop if you do. If you for sure don't smell fish while fucking her, well that is a bonus and the second sexual encounter you need to eat her out.

So the second sex encounter arrives and you have her lying naked. This time go down to her pussy, open her legs, and start kissing her pussy lips. Take both hands and gently open her lips to expose the clitoris. There is no bad fish smell, so things are looking good. It is ok however to smell a little sweat, and pussy juice. This is just normal.

Concentrate on her clit with your tongue, and then suck her clit gently. Most women will orgasm from this. Remember, to try and make her orgasm first, before you!

And another thing, on the first two to three encounters, never ask for a blow job, you must show her that you want to eat her out before a blow job ever comes up.
If she wants to suck you, she will make that move, and you then can let her. If it has been several sex encounters later and she never sucked your dick yet then you might want to start suggesting it.

My Two True Stories

Ok here are just two of my true experiences dealing with M.I.L.F and Cougars.
Towards the end you will realize why I mentioned in Chapter four to guard your heart at all cost, to not fall in love with an older woman, because it can be a heart tearing ordeal.

Story One

I was living in Las Vegas at age seventeen working at a grocery store called Von's as a courtesy clerk or box boy. Older women would seldomly hit on me, whether it was a customer or a co-worker. This one particular co- worker worked in the bread aisle every few days. Her name was Linda. She was about thirty five years of age. I had no idea she had an eye for me until a group of us box boys got together to take a ski boat out to Lake Mead for some water skiing.

Well my friends (all guys and fellow box boys) wanted to invite Linda to our day of skiing. They all thought she was very hot, and of course she was a beautiful M.I.L.F!

They invited Linda and she accepted. The day of water skiing came and it was a total of five people, four guys and one woman, Linda. It was funny, because at that time I was well reserved and quiet; not shy just quiet. All my buddies thought they were going to score with Linda, somehow, someway. I myself never imagined that it could or would happen with me.

Now keep in mind my buddies or co-workers all had hard bodies and I was a slender thin type of guy and I thought there was no chance with me compared to my buddies.
It was funny; I can remember it all, as if it was yesterday. We were on the boat, Linda was looking great in her swim suit and all three of my buddies tried hard to impress Linda that whole day. I sat back and laughed in my head as she didn't look enthused by them.

We all took turns skiing, but I tell you the hard body friends of mine kept falling like kids! It was funny. I loved to ski, so when it was my turn I stayed up the longest even jumping the wakes. This may have turned Linda on; I don't know.

Along the shore of Lake Meade would be some sandy areas to set up some towels eat and relax. We would take breaks through out that day on the sand. During one particular break I was left alone with Linda on that sandy area. While the other three took the boat real quick because they thought they had seen some sixteen year olds girls alone somewhere on the lake. They must have thought Linda was a no go and didn't want to ruin their chance picking up some dim-wit girls.

As Linda and I sat on our towels enjoying the sun, she could not stop conversating with me. All the while I was growing more excited just looking at her body glistening in the sun. We talked about work, we talked about her ex-husband who lived in California and that she had two children, I believe 8 and 6 years old staying with their dad in Cali.

We had a nice conversation, and I felt that her I knew each other like we were good friends. As the day came to an end we all went our separate ways home. I thought it was a good day.

Several days later I saw her at work working in her bread aisle. I approached her to say hi. We spoke for a while, when she asked me if I would like to go out with her to dinner. I accepted indeed. At that time I didn't have my own ride and she knew this, she would come pick me up on our dates. I lived with a room mate, and she had her own condo in a community with pool and spa.

We started a dating relationship for several months. It was about the second date we had sex and she taught me things no other girls my age ever could. Most things I know today were by Linda guiding me. Sex was amazing; she knew what she wanted, and she always initiated the sex. I spent many nights at her place. Several times at work in the back of the store, we would find a hiding spot and she would suck me off. It was great!

Our dates always consisted of adult things, not that typical young shit. We would have elegant dinners, walks, spent time in her spa with a glass of wine and much more.

I was just a senior in high school and I felt on top of the world for being with a woman like this.

One of the many things she loved was to be eaten out, and did I learn! She taught me the proper way to eat, to foreplay and many more. She particularly loved the sixty nine. I fell in love with that position too!

I grew attached to her and I knew she wanted me right back.

All was going strong and well when one night she gave me call to meet her in the parking lot of our work. It was nine o'clock at night and I waited for as he drove up to me.
I opened the passenger door and got in and asked if everything was ok. She said no.

She informed me that she was leaving town that night after she met with me to go back to California to be with her kids. She would not explain to me if she was getting back with her ex-husband.

In shock, I did not say any more or asked any more questions but one, "will I ever see you again?"

Linda could not give me a definite answer, only that she had to go back to California. We kissed and held each other for a length of time before I exited her car. We said our good byes, she drove off onto a dark road and I never saw her again.

Story Two

I was 19 when Kerry was in her early 30's to mid 30's. We met when I was working at Safeway at the deli counter. She was a customer, and soon became a regular. It seemed weekly she was coming in for a pound or two of fresh slice meat; little did I realize she ultimately wanted my meat.

She started to become more flirtatious week after week. I knew she wanted me, but I felt I could lose my job if I responded back to her flirts. I wanted her too. At this point I don't think she understood that I wanted her. I think she was looking for some kind of ice breaker or way to get me over to her place.

One particular day she asked if I had a girlfriend while I was getting her order ready. I told her I did not. She asked me if I wanted to meet her niece whom was my age. I thought, "ok sure."

"I would love to meet her" I said. Kerry wrote down her phone number and address and said to call her so she could then give me a more exact date to meet her niece.

Several days passed and I called Kerry; Kerry made the arrangements at her home to meet her niece. When I arrived at Kerry's home, she let me in but her niece was no where around. Kerry went on to tell me that her niece at the last minute got cold feet and decide not to meet me. It didn't break my heart any. Kerry said she had some dinner on the stove and asked if I would stay and eat. I did indeed.

The only people in her home were Kerry and I at that time. I couldn't tell if she lived alone or not. I did not see any pictures of other family members but yet the house was too big for one person to live in. She would not elaborate whom she lived with and I felt it was none of my business.

We had a good dinner and were finishing up with it when she asked if I wanted to go to the T.V room with her. I said yes and off we went. We sat on her couch and she turned on a movie. She sat right next to me, now I was starting to get excited. I really knew she wanted me now.

It wasn't fifteen minutes into the program when she turned and leaned in to kiss me. Of course I kissed right back. I was turned on by this M.I.L.F and I knew I was going to nail her.

She started taking her clothes off piece by piece, as I was doing the same. I was no shy guy or a virgin; I knew what I wanted to do.

She immediately went down on me and started to suck my erect cock.

Kerry knew how to deep throat, she forced my cock deep into her throat. Her mouth went all the way to the end of my shaft. I eventually put a load of my cum in the back of her throat as she gurgled it down and swallowed. .

The sex was far from over. I still had many more loads to put in her. After she swallowed me, she then stood up and grabbed my arms to stand me up off the couch. Kerry gripped my arms and told me to lay flat on my back onto the floor. With my dick still hard, she straddled me and gently inserted it deep inside her pussy. She rode and rode until she had an orgasm, she moaned a bit before she said to me, "take me and do what you want with me."

So I did just that. Although I was 19, this wasn't my first time. I told Kerry to get on her hands and knees as I got behind her to do a doggie style fuck. As I was fucking her from behind, I had my right hand wrapped around her waist to her clit and was seriously rubbing it while fucking her.

After awhile of doggie, I then told her to lie on her side and bring her knees up to the side. I love this position. I was upright on my knees while thrusting this M.I.L.F as she lay on her side. I was griping her thighs and ass cheeks as I put another load into her.

After an orgasm, I laid down next to her as she thanked me for the sex. Few minutes went by and she started to get dress, as I did to. I did not want to be too intrusive so I thanked her for the nice evening and asked if I could see her again. She said that might be possible and she would come find me. And yes - her wanting me to meet her niece was all made up hoax by Kerry.

I continued my life as normal, but I never did see Kerry come back to the deli to order her meat.